RADIANT RENEWAL

Transforming Menopause into a Journey of Self-Discovery and Success

Perry S. Ferraro

TABLE OF CONTENTS

INTRODUCTION

Understanding menopause

By the end of the next several years, 1.1 billion women are expected to have experienced menopause. Women in their prime, running their own businesses, households, and even countries. Even though for around half of the population, menopause is a normal transition in life, the subject of menopause is sometimes shrouded in shame and fear of criticism – about ageing, attractiveness, fertility, and even professional usefulness. The silence that too many women experience is inherited from generation to generation.

It's time to change the perception of menopause from something to be feared to one that offers great potential for self-care, personal development, and a period when life may be satisfying. Each woman's experience is as distinct as she is, ranging from the downright dismal to the uplifted, and it breaks the silence surrounding this long misunderstood life stage.

We hope these pages will reassure you that you are not alone and provide you the opportunity to seek the support you may need if you are currently going through menopause, are concerned that you will go through menopause, or know someone who is. Why not tell individuals who are dear to you that you are going through menopause? It might even give you the confidence to talk about your personal experiences. We can eliminate the stigma associated with menopause one story at a time.

Everything in our body is regulated by hormones, including our sexuality, energy levels, and mood. Therefore, it should come as no surprise that changes brought on by menopause may affect how we connect with others. The vibrations of this transition often reach our loved ones before we do. Close friends may sense an emotional shift, spouses may note a change in desire, and children may observe mood swings.

Low mood and anxiety, two common menopausal symptoms, might develop gradually to the point that we are oblivious to them. A problem may arise because intimacy may become less appealing as a result of physical changes at home. The effects of fatigue and a crippling loss of confidence at work can be detrimental to professional performance.

Women don't talk enough about the changes they are going through, which breeds isolation. Additionally, loved ones may experience difficulties. According to one survey, 38% of partners feel powerless to support their partners through menopause, which causes arguments in one-third of marriages.

Women's own experiences show how important it is to discuss the emotional effects of midlife hormone changes so that all women going through menopause can get the support they need.

53-year-old Lisa faced menopause head-on and won the battle. She entered this new phase of her life with a positive outlook and a desire to advance herself. Lisa took proactive steps to lessen her symptoms as soon as she became aware of the changes her body would experience throughout menopause. Yoga and meditation became her partners as she maintained her balance and energy through regular exercise.

Lisa prioritized looking for herself. She focused on eating well and drinking plenty of water. She also asked her friends and family for assistance, disclosing her problems with them and receiving counsel from them.

Lisa focused on her hobbies rather than the challenges. She rekindled her love of painting and enrolled in an art class, where she gained fulfilment in using vivid colors to express herself.

Throughout her menopause experience, Lisa stayed in touch with her inner self. She recognized and appreciated her shifting body as a sign of power and wisdom. She bravely pursued her aspirations, showing others that age is no impediment to success. Lisa developed persistence and desire as a result of her experiences. She emerged from menopause stronger, inspiring those around her with her zest for life and upbeat outlook.

PART 1

Exploring the biology and hormonal changes during menopause

Menopause has traditionally been regarded as a precursor to death, a transformation from woman to crone with her exit ticket already punched. This is due to the fact that a woman's worth was determined by her reproductive capabilities, and hence her femininity, as defined by a narrow, patriarchal standard.

Menopause medical terminology presently reflects this cliché. For example, it is usual to describe that during menopause, the ovarian supply of eggs is "exhausted," but the term of failure or tiredness is never used.

Many young girls who had no knowledge of puberty awoke one morning drenched in blood from their first period, scared that they were dying. In the 1940s, this was my mother's experience. For many women, menopause is a reflection of this, with a slew of unexpected symptoms that they may be reluctant to address openly.

We can do better if we embrace the concept of a feminist menopause. Women ought to be able to experience these changes in their bodies with facts and without fear, shame, or concealment. A feminist menopause rejects the patriarchal assumption that a woman's worth is linked to her ovarian function and that the end of her reproductive life is the end of her productive life. The medical community should provide significantly more information to women about how their hormones change in middle age, what to expect, and what may be treated medically.

The term "menopause" is derived from the Greek words for month and cessation, and refers to the last menstrual period. In actuality, menopause is a puberty-like transition of hormonal changes that leads from one biological period of life to another. Menopause is caused by changes in the ovaries as well as the brain. Women are born with a limited amount of eggs, or oocytes, and decades of ovulation reduce oocyte availability and quality, influencing oestrogen and progesterone production as well as the brain's sensitivity to these chemicals. This period is known medically as the menopause transition. These hormonal changes often begin in a woman's mid-40s and can linger for years, causing symptoms such as irregular menstruation, hot flushes (or flashes), vaginal dryness, depression, difficulty sleeping, and brain fog.

A woman eventually gets her last menstrual period, which is widely regarded as the onset of menopause. However, that incident has just a minor impact on the process. The last menstrual period is critical for determining whether to discontinue contraception, and its arrival can influence how clinicians assess irregular menstrual flow. But what actually matters for people with ovaries begins years before the last menstrual period and lasts a lifetime, as the hormonal changes of the transition can increase women's risk of illnesses such as heart disease, stroke, dementia, and osteoporosis. Of course, women may be relieved when their monthly pains, heavy or irregular periods, or anxieties of unexpected pregnancies are over.

Many women, however, are unaware of the basic biology of menopause and are unsure what to expect when they no longer have a monthly menstruation. They may be concerned that a hot-flush inferno will leave them dripping with sweat at work, or they may be apprehensive about discussing vaginal dryness with their sexual partner. What lady wants to accept that she now plays for a squad deemed insignificant by society? When you consider that much of menopause occurs "down there," the information gap is unsurprising.

Women may fail to communicate uncomfortable symptoms with a medical professional because they mistakenly believe there are no safe, effective treatments. As a physician and author who frequently publishes and speaks about women's health, I've heard from many women who thought their doctors were unable or unwilling to answer their queries about changes in their bodies. They've described being disregarded with blank glances or platitudes like "It's not that bad" or "That's just part of being a woman," or being urged to return when they're "really in menopause." the knowledge gap is so wide that many women are unsure of these signs of age. Are they in it or out of it? This confusion can be traced back to the misplaced emphasis on the last menstrual period, as well as the use of confusing terminology: the menopause transition, or the time leading up to the final menstrual period, is frequently referred to as perimenopause; perimenopause describes the menopause transition plus the first year without a period. However, because there is no last call announcing the last menstrual period, a woman is termed postmenopausal (or often just "in menopause") after a year without a period. Because the last period has little impact on how we manage the majority of the menopause experience, it's usual to refer to the entire process as menopause.

It's understandable that relying on missing periods for a diagnosis can be annoying, so it's no wonder that a variety of companies are now selling tests that claim to identify a woman where she is in her menopausal transition. However, no one blood, saliva, or urine test can reliably indicate whether or not a woman is nearing the end of her menstrual cycle. The hormonal instability of the menopausal transition is so severe that hormone levels may indicate menopause one month and be normal two months later. These tests are mainly worthless because they provide a snapshot of continually changing hormone levels, and treatment for problematic symptoms is not dependent on hormone levels. These diagnostics essentially profit by exploiting inadequacies in medicine.

Over the last two decades, there has been a flood of interesting new menopause research. Scientists have discovered that certain antidepressants and other treatments can help to minimize hot flushes. Hormonal therapy can help with menopausal genitourinary symptoms (vaginal dryness and pain during sex). According to research, brain fog exists – but it is only transitory. We are living in a medical menopausal renaissance, yet many women are not reaping the benefits.

As a result, women seeking information may turn to sources that appear to be educated but, coincidentally, frequently promote items — many of which are unproven and even hazardous — to cure menopausal symptoms. As a result, there is a burgeoning industry for over-the-counter remedies promoted to menopausal women and promising help from symptoms such as hot flashes and sleep issues, many with little supporting data. Supplements are not tested for safety in the United States, and some "menopause supplements" contain chemicals that are either not proven to aid with symptoms or may cause actual harm.

A burgeoning industry exists for compounded, so-called bioidentical hormones. These products are not subject to proper regulatory scrutiny, and a recent assessment from the National Academies of Sciences, Engineering, and Medicine determined that there is little evidence available concerning their safety and effectiveness. Personally, I only use oestrogen that has been approved by the Food and Drug Administration. I want to know exactly what my body is ingesting, and a compounded medication simply cannot provide that precision and safety. The fact that many women feel more at ease taking products that are not indicated by menopause experts speaks much about communication gaps in medicine as well as those who prey on women. These gaps are particularly concerning given that science is not lacking.

Western medicine has already developed methods for informing patients about important hormonal shifts. After all, pediatricians often discuss puberty with their patients during annual visits, and their discussions are tailored to age and symptoms. Doctors should have comparable conversations with late-thirties women so that their patients are prepared. Menstrual abnormalities, hot flushes, sadness, and brain fog can begin several years before a woman's final menstrual period, which usually occurs in her early 50s. These discussions can also motivate women to take steps to protect their health throughout menopause, such as increasing activity and ensuring enough calcium intake.

For far too long, women have had to fight to understand the truth about menopause, to fight for their health and sanity. Speaking up about a female body's worries as it ages should be regarded normal, not daring.

Menopause isn't the end of the world. We must eradicate the sexist belief that a woman's worth is determined by her oestrogen and age. Instead, consider menopause to be a new stage in life, with the previous stage serving as a milestone along the road. When women need assistance navigating their symptoms and the health consequences of menopause, they should have access to clear, non-sexist information and effective solutions. Eventually, accessing menopause treatment will not need an act of feminism, but that will never happen if we remain silent.

Menopause myths and misunderstandings debunked

It's a common feeling of moving on in life that all women have had throughout history. Yet, in many cultures around the world, society concentrates on the hardships of menopause rather than on it as a milestone that ushers in a new phase of confidence and leadership.

As a result, many myths and misconceptions about menopause continue, requiring women and those around them to sort fact from fiction in order to understand this life phase. Here are five of the most common beliefs about menopause, along with the facts to dispel them.

Myth #1: Menopause begins when a woman's period stops.

Menopause is the irreversible cessation of menstruation and thus fertility. Menopause is diagnosed after a woman has gone a year without having a period. Many of the symptoms frequently associated with menopause occur during perimenopause (also known as the menopausal transition), which refers to the years preceding and following the final menstrual period. The length of perimenopause before the last menstrual period varies substantially. Oestrogen and progesterone levels fluctuate dramatically during perimenopause. These changes are assumed to be the source of menopausal symptoms in many women in their 40s. Following the menopausal transition, which typically lasts four years, women enter the postmenopauses phase, which refers to the time following the last menstrual period.

The typical age for menopause in the United States is around 50 to 51. Menopause, on the other hand, is not uncommon in women aged 45 to 55. When menopause happens before the age of 40, it is considered premature. Premature menopause is also known as primary ovarian insufficiency or premature ovarian failure.

Myth #2: Hot flashes are the only menopausal symptom.

The majority of symptoms occur during perimenopause and early postmenopause, with approximately 75% of women suffering hot flashes—which some women refer to as power surges. During a hot flash, the temperature regulating Centre of the brain malfunctions, causing blood vessels near the skin's surface to expand and increase blood flow. Women will feel warm or heated as a result, and perspiration may be profuse. Another typical symptom is difficulty sleeping, which can occur when a hot flash causes a woman to wake up in the middle of the night. Even if they are not having a hot flash, women may have difficulty sleeping. Other symptoms include mood swings and sensations of forgetfulness. Many women may find it beneficial to look to their mothers' and sisters' experiences to better understand what to expect as they approach perimenopause. Vaginal dryness or uncomfortable intercourse may occur in some women.

Myth #3: Menopause causes a decline in sexual desire.

Many women suffer a reduction in libido as they age, but it is difficult to define what constitutes normal sex drive and which factors have the most influence on sexual desire. There has been no conclusive research on whether ageing or hormone changes are the most important causes. Other menopausal symptoms, such as mood changes, sleep difficulty, or vaginal dryness, may also have an impact on sexual function. When these difficulties are addressed, many women's sexual function improves.

Myth #4: Menopause is incurable.

Menopause is not an illness, despite how it is frequently portrayed or addressed. It is a normal process. Women can, however, take actions to alleviate some of the symptoms of menopause, starting with maintaining appropriate sleep habits, altering clothes and room temperature to keep cooler, and controlling stress. Nonhormonal therapy and cooling equipment, in addition to lifestyle adjustments, may be beneficial. Lubricants and vaginal moisturizers are quite beneficial for vaginal dryness. Medications may also help with common menopausal symptoms. If nonhormonal approaches have failed to relieve symptoms such as hot flashes and vaginal dryness, hormone therapy may be a useful option.

As women reach their mid-40s or begin to experience monthly irregularity or menopausal symptoms, it's critical to talk to their doctor about what to expect and how to manage symptoms. The best place to start is with primary care providers and gynecologists who are familiar with menopause. If a woman's symptoms are severe and difficult to cure, or if she has other medical issues such as diabetes, a family history of breast cancer, or migraine headaches, she should consult a menopausal specialist.

Myth #5: Menopause has no advantages.

As Margaret Mead shows out, there are enormous benefits to being postmenopausal. Many women are relieved to be free of pregnancy prevention and menstrual cycles. Many women also notice that premenstrual symptoms including bloating, migraine headaches, and premenstrual mood fluctuations diminish dramatically as they reach menopause.

Accepting menopause as a life-changing experience

Menopause, sometimes known as the "change of life," is a normal and transforming stage in a woman's life. Instead than considering menopause as a negative experience, let us see it as a woman's Second Spring—a period of growth, wisdom, and fresh freedom. In this article, we will look at how botanicals and CBD can help with menopause symptoms, and how taking a holistic approach can help us face this challenge with grace, fortitude, and renewed vigour.

A woman's second spring, also known as peri/menopause, is a natural biological event that marks the end of her reproductive years. Menopause, like spring, provides women with opportunities for self-reflection and personal growth. Accepting this shift with optimism can make it easier to bear and allow us to celebrate the wisdom, strength, and confidence that come with this period of life. Nature can also provide assistance.

For generations, nature's nurturers, botanicals, or herbal treatments, have been utilized to support women during menopause. The following botanicals were chosen for their separate qualities as well as their synergistic effect in Menopause Balance.

• Black Cohosh balances oestrogen levels in your body, boosting or reducing this vital hormone according to your body's demands. It can provide relief and comfort by reducing hot flashes and nocturnal sweats.

• Wild Yam balances the use and function of oestrogen and progesterone in the body.

• Alfalfa provides the body with immune-boosting phytosterols and critical minerals that are commonly lacking when hormones are out of whack.

• Lemon Balm relaxes and calms stressed bodies while balancing hormones to help with mood, focus, sleep, and digestion.

• Maca provides the body with the ability to adapt to stress and anxiety while also revitalizing the immune system, sexual functions, and energy levels.

• CBD promotes the body's inherent anti-inflammatory qualities.

Night Sky is a proprietary blend of CBD and carefully selected, clean, and strong botanicals designed to calm a restless mind and promote deep, restorative sleep.

• Albizzia has a mild sedative effect that helps with sleep and anxiety, reduces inflammation, and can aid with depression and other mood concerns.

• California Poppy has a sedative effect that promotes sleep, relieves anxiety and tension, and improves brain function.

• Chinese knotweed contains antioxidants and may aid in the treatment of sleep disorders and nerve illnesses.

• Passion Flower soothes sleep difficulties and creates an overall soothing effect, which aids in the reduction of anxiety and tension.

• Spiny Zizyphus improves sleep, has anti-inflammatory qualities, and is believed to calm the brain and nervous system.

• Reishi Mushroom revitalizes your body and calms sleep disturbances, aids in the resolution of digestive issues, and aids in the relaxation of your body in response to daily tensions.

• Rosacea aids digestion and is believed to affect the heart, liver, and spleen.

• Radish Seed is used to alleviate digestive problems and stomach pain.

• CBD promotes the body's inherent anti-inflammatory characteristics, as well as digestion and immunological function. It also helps with sleep, tension, and anxiety alleviation. CBD has been used to help people sleep better.

In addition to using Respect Wellness products, you can assist your transformation by including daily mind-body practices. Mindfulness is a practice in which you quiet your mind via meditation to assist manage stress, create emotional balance, and increase self-awareness. Yoga can enhance flexibility, reduce muscle tension, and promote relaxation. Embracing creativity in the form of art, writing, and/or music can be a means of self-expression and personal development. During menopause, a well-balanced and healthy diet is essential. Including nutrient-dense, nutritious protein-rich foods like fruits, vegetables, whole grains, and healthy fats in your diet might help you feel better overall.

Menopause is a new beginning, not an end, in a woman's life—a Second Spring. We may welcome these changes while enjoying the knowledge and resilience that come with them by taking a holistic approach that integrates Respect Wellness's botanicals with CBD and your choice of mind-body practices. Menopause is a period of self-discovery and development. Allow grace to be your guiding light on this transformative path.

PART 2: Navigating Physical Changes: Caring for Your Body

Managing common symptoms like hot flashes, night sweats, and weight changes

While the average age is 51, the majority of women will experience menopause between the ages of 40 and 58. Perimenopause is a transition stage during which you may experience menopausal symptoms but continue to have a monthly cycle. Perimenopause symptoms can appear up to seven years before the end of the menstrual cycle.

Menopause happens before the age of 40. If you believe you are going through early menopause, talk to your doctor about hormone replacement treatment to help avoid cardiovascular disease and bone health.

How can you tell if you're in menopause?

Going a year without a monthly cycle is the most telling sign that you're in menopause.

What are the physical symptoms of menopause?

Hot flashes, nocturnal sweats, vaginal dryness, hair loss, weight gain (particularly around the stomach), skin changes, arthralgia (joint pain), sleep disruption, and muscle tone loss are also frequent symptoms. But you don't have to put up with the discomfort. There are therapeutic alternatives available, including lifestyle changes that can help alleviate annoying symptoms. I ask my patients about their most annoying symptoms, and we discuss ways to manage them so they can feel better.

What can be done to reduce the weight gain associated with menopause?

There are methods for reducing weight gain during menopause. Begin adopting healthy lifestyle practices before menopause by exercising and eating well to establish positive habits. Ageing is connected with metabolic changes, muscular loss, and a rise in body fat. We become less physically active as we age, which contributes significantly to weight gain. Weight gain around the waist raises the risk of diabetes, high cholesterol, cardiovascular disease, osteoarthritis, and some cancers (breast, uterine, and colon). Weight gain, in addition to having a detrimental influence on health, frequently leads to poor self-image and melancholy.

Adhering to a nutritious diet and engaging in regular physical activity is critical to your overall health and well-being. A healthy diet includes controlling portion sizes and reducing sugar, processed carbs, fat, and processed foods. The Mediterranean diet has been demonstrated to aid in weight loss, improve cognition, reduce the risk of dementia and osteoporosis, and improve cardiovascular health. Walking, Pilates, and yoga are weight-bearing workouts that help preserve posture, balance, and core strength.

Furthermore, stress and mental wellbeing must be managed because stress might exacerbate other menopausal symptoms. Stress can be managed with cognitive behavioral therapy. Pilates, acupuncture, and yoga, for example, can help people quiet their brain and nervous system, tune in to their breathing, and be mindful of the present moment. People who practice these healthy practices maintain better control of their weight and overall health during the menopause transition.

How does a hot flash feel?

Hot flashes are commonly described as a sudden feeling of warmth, usually from the nipple line up, accompanied by sweating. During hot flashes, some people report an increase in heart rate. Night sweats are hot flashes that occur while sleeping, frequently resulting in sweating bouts that are strong enough to soak through clothing and bedding. Hot flashes and night sweats can range in severity and frequency from mild to severe.

What causes nocturnal sweats and hot flashes?

Because hormonal changes affect the way your brain regulates body heat, hot flashes and nocturnal sweats occur during perimenopause and menopause. It's unclear why some women have stronger vasomotor symptoms (hot flashes and night sweats) than others throughout menopause.

When should I be concerned about night sweats and hot flashes?

If hot flashes and night sweats are interfering with your quality of life, consult your doctor. Behavioral therapy, non-hormonal medicines, and hormone therapy are all possible therapeutic choices.

Is hair loss caused by menopause?

Menopause-related hormonal changes might contribute to hair loss. The most prevalent causes of telogen effluvium, or unexpected rapid hair loss, include stress and shifting hormones during the menopause transition. Female pattern baldness is also frequent. Because hormones have a role, it is more common after menopause. Hair loss can be influenced by underlying medical issues, genes, and particular style practices.

Maintain a healthy diet to help prevent hair loss. Certain supplements (iron, zinc, vitamins D and B) may be beneficial. Be gentle with your hair and follicles as well. Hairstyles that create pulling should be avoided. Avoid using direct heat on your hair and maintain it well-conditioned. Natural oils such as argan oil, Jamaican black castor oil, and olive oil may be beneficial. Over-the-counter medicines such as minoxidil or laser caps or helmets may help. Any of these therapies can take up to four months to work. If there hasn't been any improvement after four months, it's time to see a doctor. Hormone replacement treatment has been demonstrated to benefit some ladies suffering from hair loss.

Is it true that menopause causes emotional changes as well?

Yes. Emotional symptoms might appear as early as the perimenopause. Memory problems (sometimes referred to as "brain fog"), impatience, mood fluctuations, increased anxiety, and sadness are all common symptoms. These symptoms frequently create severe distress and can harm personal and professional relationships. According to some patients, the emotional toll is the most difficult. A history of depression or anxiety illness increases the likelihood of symptom recurrence or worsening during the menopause transition. Exercise, relaxation techniques, and dietary adjustments can all be beneficial. Seeing a therapist and potentially taking medication such as mood stabilizers or hormone replacement treatment can help people having severe symptoms.

What effect does menopause have on sex?

The decrease of oestrogen during menopause can cause vaginal tissues to become thinner, dryer, and less flexible. This can cause vaginal discomfort and uncomfortable intercourse, limiting one's ability to become aroused and enjoy intercourse. Unlike other menopausal symptoms, which improve with time, vaginal difficulties might deteriorate if left untreated. Furthermore, women in their forties and fifties frequently report of diminished sex drive and trouble achieving orgasm. Non-hormonal and hormonal treatment alternatives that are both safe and effective are available. Pelvic floor physical treatment and sex therapy can be beneficial in some circumstances. Along with vaginal oestrogen therapies, the UChicago Woman Lab website offers information on vaginal moisturizers, lubricants, and pelvic floor physical therapy.

Menopause lasts how long?

Most people's symptoms improve over time. It normally takes four to five years from the last menstrual period. Researchers aren't sure why, but symptoms stay longer for particular ethnicities, such as Black Americans, and are generally seen as more bothersome. Your quality of life should not be jeopardized. When lifestyle changes do not alleviate menopausal symptoms, your doctor can recommend alternative treatments.

Are menopause supplements effective?

Many over-the-counter supplements are claimed to aid with hot flashes and night sweats, including black cohosh, chaste berry, evening primrose oil, and soy. However, there is little evidence to back up their claims of benefit. The majority of research have found them to be no more effective than placebos. Please with your doctor before beginning any supplements to ensure that they are safe and do not interact with any drugs you are taking.

Tips for promoting hormonal balance with nutrition and diet

It can be challenging to maintain hormonal balance while using drugs. Doctor-prescribed medications are appropriate for those women who have severe hormonal abnormalities. Most women, on the other hand, do not require such rigorous treatment for hormone imbalance. These ladies can eat items that assist the body naturally produce the necessary hormones.

Let's have a look at some foods that have been shown to naturally improve hormonal dysregulation and balance hormones:

Flaxseeds are a type of seed. Flaxseeds tend to be beneficial to PCOS women. Taking flaxseeds improves metabolic factors, leading to more weight loss and higher fertility.

Broccoli is a vegetable. Broccoli and other Brassica family members have been shown to improve liver health and lower the risk of metabolic liver disease. This can assist ladies suffering from PCOS in balancing their hormones. Furthermore, broccoli consumption can aid in the restoration of the gut microbiome, which enhances metabolic health.

• Avocadoes. Avocados contain a lot of monounsaturated fats. They can reduce your risk of heart disease by lowering your cholesterol and triglycerides. They can aid in the reduction of inflammation and the normal production of hormones.

• Sailfish. Salmon is high in omega-3 fatty acids, which are important for many aspects of health. Salmon and other low-mercury fish have protein that increases satiety without causing blood sugar swings.

Quinoa is a grain. Quinoa can help to balance hormones by lowering blood sugar levels, boosting lipid profiles, and reducing belly fat. These are significant benefits that have the potential to enhance PCOS symptoms and results.

Spinach is a vegetable. Spinach and other leafy greens are high in phytonutrients. Spinach can help women with PCOS lose belly fat and improve their metabolic profile, resulting in better hormone balance.

• Cashews. Women can enjoy almonds as a healthy snack. They lower blood sugar swings and inhibit hunger without causing weight gain.

Chia seeds are a type of seed. Chia seeds are high in fibre because they absorb water, allowing for better GI function. They may have an anti-inflammatory impact and may improve blood pressure management when consumed. Chia seeds can also assist to reduce blood sugar swings.

• Turkey is a country. Tryptophan is an amino acid precursor in the formation of several essential mood and appetite neurotransmitters found in turkey. When these neurotransmitters are in balance, you may have better sleep and less hunger.

• Blueberries are delicious. Blueberries are abundant in antioxidants, which help to minimize cell stress. They've been demonstrated to boost both female and male fertility.

• Extra virgin olive oil. Olive oil is high in polyunsaturated fats, which aid to reduce inflammation and belly obesity. It has been demonstrated that it is toxic to breast cancer cells, which may imply that it improves hormone balance in women with estrogen-sensitive malignancies such as breast cancer.

• Legumes. Lentils have a high fiber content and are a good source of starch. They lessen blood sugar fluctuations, reduce abdominal fat, and protect the gut microbiota. These can aid in the restoration of your body's natural hormone levels.

• Yoghurt from Greece. Yoghurt is a fermented food that includes beneficial probiotic bacteria. This improves your gut microbiota and promotes natural hormone repair.

• A cup of green tea. Green tea has a lot of antioxidants, which helps with cellular health. Green tea can assist women with PCOS lower insulin resistance and improve metabolism.

Pomegranates are a type of fruit. These are abundant in antioxidants and help to keep blood sugar and abdominal fat in check. They may be useful in resolving inflammatory conditions that impair normal hormonal balance.

• Eggs. Eggs are high in protein and contain choline, which is beneficial to brain health. Eggs also help to decrease appetite and aid in weight loss by keeping you satisfied for longer.

• Tofu. Tofu contains a lot of soy isoflavones. Because they contain very little additional fat, they assist balance female hormones in menopausal women and promote lower body fat levels. This alone can help PCOS women achieve more balanced hormone levels.

• Foods that have been fermented. Fermented foods such as yoghurt, miso, tempeh, sauerkraut, and kimchi provide beneficial probiotics that improve intestinal health. A healthy gut means reduced inflammation and better hormonal balances.

• Cinnamon is a spice. Cinnamon comes in a variety of forms. The majority of them include coumarin, which contributes to their anti-inflammatory qualities. It helps to stabilize blood sugar, stimulates weight loss, and lowers lipid levels.

In general, lowering inflammation creates a better environment for minimizing stress on your body's cells. This allows your hormones to balance normally. Reduced body fat means improved hormone levels and fewer symptoms in women with PCOS.

While most meals are safe to consume in moderation, the foods that may benefit your unique illness may not be the same as those that will benefit another individual with comparable concerns. Because balancing hormones through diet can be complicated, you should seek the assistance of your healthcare practitioner or a hormone health nutritionist to help you manage your specific circumstances.

Exercise and fitness routines for staying fit and healthy

The most vital, uncontroversial, and straightforward thing that everyone can and should do is exercise. The advantages are as follows:

A. Exercise improves cardiovascular and respiratory function. It decreases the metabolic hazards linked with decreased oestrogen when done on a regular basis. It raises HDL while decreasing LDL, triglycerides, and fibrinogen. Another advantage is a lower risk of high blood pressure, heart attacks, and strokes.

b. Exercise can aid in the creation of a calorie deficit and the reduction of midlife weight gain.

c. It promotes bone mass. Strength training and impact activities (such as walking or running) can help to counteract bone mineral density decrease and prevent osteoporosis.

d. It also helps with low back discomfort.

e. It has been shown to help relieve stress and boost mood.

f. It may help to minimize hot flashes and hence the "Domino effect."

Although there was no definitive evidence from randomized controlled trials on whether exercise is an effective treatment for lowering hot flushes and night sweats in menopausal women, the most recent Cochrane review did identify a modest tendency that exercise was more beneficial than no intervention.

How to Get Started

It's never too late to start working out. The idea is to begin cautiously and do activities that you enjoy, such as walking, cycling, vigorous garden work, swimming, cardio machines or group fitness programmes. Regular exercise can help to improve one's general well-being. Even mild physical activity, such as simply moving the body enough to get the heart pounding, provides numerous health benefits, including increased energy. The action should be brisk enough to get the heart pounding but not so fast that you are out of breath or weary.

To get the maximal heart rate during exercise, subtract the woman's age from 220. Multiply the maximal heart rate by 50/100 and 80/100 to achieve the ideal heart rate range. During the first few weeks of a fitness programme, aim for the lowest part of the target zone (50 percent). Gradually progress to the upper half of the goal zone (75%). After six months or more of consistent exercise, one may be able to exercise at up to 85 percent of one's maximal heart rate comfortably.

Women taking hypertension medications should be aware that only a few high blood pressure medications, particularly beta blockers, lower the maximum heart rate and consequently the target zone rate. Such ladies should consult their doctors to determine whether they need to adopt a lower target heart rate.

The talk test is a practical method for tracking exercise intensity. Moderate intensity activity, such as strolling at 3.5

mph, allows a lady to chat but not sing and should not leave her out of breath. She should be able to speak a few words but not carry on a conversation during strong aerobic exercise, such as step aerobics. Exercise at the target heart rate improves fitness and conditions the lungs, heart, circulation, and muscles.

EXERCISES OF DIFFERENCE

The following exercises can aid in the development and maintenance of bone density and mass:

Weight-bearing, high-impact workouts include dancing, high-intensity aerobics, running / jogging, jumping rope, stair climbing, and sports such as tennis, basketball, volleyball, or gymnastics. These are best suited for people who are not osteoporotic, have low bone mass, and are not fragile.

Walking (treadmill or outside), elliptical training machines, stair steppers, and low impact aerobics are examples of weight bearing, low impact activities. Women who cannot conduct high-impact workouts may prefer this group of activities to develop bones.

Lifting weights, using elastic bands or weight machines for exercise, and using simple functional actions such as standing or lifting one's own body weight are all examples of weight or strength training or resistance training exercises.

Cycling, swimming, stretching, and flexibility exercises are examples of nonweight bearing, nonimpact activities. These should be incorporated into a thorough fitness programme. These alone do not contribute to bone formation.

Non-impact activities: Include exercises that aid with posture and attitude balance, such as T'ai Chi.

Menopause-friendly exercise prescription: A postmenopausal woman's exercise programme should contain endurance (aerobic), strength, and balance exercises. Aerobics, weight bearing, and resistance activities are all beneficial for increasing bone mineral density in postmenopausal women.

Resistance and weight bearing exercise three days a week (on alternate days) may be an effective workout prescription. It is important to rotate the exercise for all muscle groups, preferably with a trainer. On the remaining days of the week, brisk walking at a speed of five to six kilometres per hour, cycling, treadmill, gardening, or dancing may be done.

Warming up before exercise can help to reduce exercise-related injuries and pain afterward. Aim for two hours and thirty minutes of moderate aerobic activity each week. Other deep breathing, yoga, and stretching techniques can help with stress management and menopausal symptoms.

Step-By-Step Approach

Step 1: Warm up by stretching, walking on a treadmill for five minutes, or going for a brisk walk. Because the body becomes less flexible as we age, it is critical to warm up before working exercise.

Step 2: Perform aerobic exercise that raises the heart rate and burns fat. Taking a dancing class, an aerobics class, going for a run or a bike ride, enrolling in kickboxing, or spending time on an elliptical machine all benefit the big muscle groups and improve cardiovascular function.

Step 3: To maintain your bones healthy, lift weights, utilize resistance bands, or try body weight strength training. Menopause is a common time for women to lose bone density, often known as osteoporosis. They must help keep their bones robust by keeping their muscles strong. Strength exercise can also aid to fire up the slowing metabolism and burn fat even while resting, so avoiding the dreaded menopausal weight gain.

Step 4: Improve your flexibility by doing routines that stretch your muscles, such as yoga and Pilates. This can improve muscle function. Each night, the lady must devote time to yoga and meditation in order to alleviate some of the worry that is a common symptom of menopause.

Step 5: Cool down after an exercise by walking for a few minutes and stretching to reduce any soreness caused by a particularly strenuous workout. This provides the body a chance to relax and promotes normal breathing and a slowing of the heart rate when one finishes exercising for a healthy end to this menopause friendly activity.

The finest routine

A routine of twice a day calcium citrate supplementation (800 mg) plus resistance exercise three times a week enhances bone density in postmenopausal women, whether or not the women is taking estrogen. The risk of osteoporosis in the generally sensitive areas of the spine and hip can be minimized by taking simple efforts such as consuming a balanced diet with lots of calcium and Vitamin D and in weight bearing exercise.

1. Wall or smith squat

2. Pull down on the lats

3. Leg extension

4. Military press with one arm

5. Row of seated people

6. Back elongation

The following are descriptions of a few key exercises:

A squat

The squat is one of the best exercises for developing and displaying raw strength. Place a couple iron plates on the bar, cross your shoulders, squat until your thighs are parallel to the ground, and then stand back up. It may appear simple, yet it is one of the most intensive workouts for building bone density. Although many recreational lifters prefer a greater rep range, alternating between moderate and heavy lifting of six to eight and four to six reps yields the best results.

The shoulder press

Another spectacular strength exhibition is the shoulder press, which involves raising a barbell straight over your head. The shoulder press is also one of the workouts that has the greatest impact on bone density. Although completing dumbbell shoulder lifts helps to develop the stabilizer muscles. When it comes to bone density, weight is everything, so select a shoulder press station or a power cage and utilize a barbell.

Pull down on the lats

Lat pull downs work the lats, biceps, and forearms. A good stretch in the lats, right under the arms, should be felt at the top of the action. When one is strong enough, they can progress to pull ups and even weighted pull ups.

Leg extension

The leg press allows you to evaluate the genuine strength of your quadriceps, hamstrings, glutes, and calves without having to worry about your balance or lower back. This exercise can move a lot of weight, and the tension causes an increase in bone mineral density.

Row of seated people

The seated row works the same muscles as the lat pull-down, but it additionally engages the lower back and glutes as stabilizers and targets the traps. The key to performing this exercise safely is to not sway as you move. The buttocks should lock the body into a comfortable hip angle that does not fluctuate.

At least seven to ten minutes of cardiovascular weight-bearing activity, such as weighted walking, stair climbing, and jogging, are included in each training session, and small muscle group workouts employing thera-bands and physio-balls fill out the study routine. The intensity of the weight-bearing activity and the level of resistance training are critical to reaching the goal of enhanced bone health. Success requires gradually increasing the weight lifted and consistently training two to three times each week.

Tai chi

This is the most often used balance exercise. Yin (receptive) and yang (active) principles are claimed to be physically and energetically balanced through T'ai Chi Ch'uan techniques: 'From ultimate softness comes ultimate hardness.'

The core training consists of two primary components: the solo form, a slow sequence of movements emphasizing a straight spine, relaxed breathing, and a natural range of motion; and different styles of pushing hands, for training reflex sensitivity through various motions from the forms, in concert with a training partner, in order to learn leverage, timing, coordination, and positioning when interacting with another.

Participants are taught not to fight or resist an incoming force, but rather to meet it softly and 'stick' to it, following its motion and remaining in physical contact until the incoming force of attack exhausts itself or can be safely redirected as a result of meeting yang with yin. The major purpose of T'ai Chi Ch'uan training is to achieve this yin/yang or yang/yin balance in battle (and, by extension, other areas of one's life). 'The soft and flexible will vanquish the harsh and strong.' Kindness is also emphasized in traditional schools. One is expected to be merciful to one's adversaries.

T'ai chi training may benefit patients with osteoarthritis by strengthening joint musculature and increasing range of motion and flexibility, and it may be used in addition to traditional treatment.

Exercise's effect on bone mineral density

When the muscles that link to the bones strengthen, the bones get stronger. Bone changes occur at a considerably slower rate than strength changes. Compound workout routines with high load and low reps encourage muscle development around the hips, spine, and arms, building bone strength in those vulnerable places and throughout the body. Even if BMD is not improved as evaluated by the dexascan, resistance training of sufficient intensity will significantly reduce lifetime fracture risk.

The maximum load, not the load frequency, is most important in BMD alterations. It is advisable to use a limited number of loading cycles. The spine's trabecular bone remodels faster than the cortical bones of the hip and wrist. The intensity with which the activity is conducted correlates directly with the increase in BMD. Under ideal conditions, bone remodeling can take four to six months or more, and the quantitative effects of exercise may not be visible for years. BMD increases, on the other hand, have been documented with only five resistance exercises, hip extension, knee extension, lateral pull-down, back extension, and abdominal flexion (3 8 at 80% 1RM) twice a week for a year.

The Indian Council of Medical Research (ICMR) reported a considerable center wise disparity in BMD in India. The paradox of reduced fracture rates among IndoAsian women compared to Caucasian women has also been highlighted, despite the former group having lesser bone mass at maturity. This has raised the possibility of detecting bone mineral apparent density (BMAD) in Indian women.

What to avoid

Although all postmenopausal women should be encouraged to engage in lifestyle practices that reduce the risk of bone loss and osteoporotic fractures, these exercises for women with osteoporosis should not include high-impact aerobics or activities that are likely to result in a fall, such as exercising on slippery floors or step aerobics. Activities that require frequent or resisted trunk flexion, such as sit-ups or toe touches, should also be avoided due to the higher loads exerted on the spine, which may result in spine fracture.

Another thing to consider is when to quit exercising. This is a serious warning to all women. Senior women should be able to read their bodies' signals. It is critical not to disregard the signs of overwork, which can lead to serious problems such as heart attack and damage. If you have a problem when exercising, it is best to pause and adjust your workouts.

Excessive activity should also be avoided if proper caloric and protein intake is not met.

When should they refrain from exercising? Certain medical issues make exercising impossible. These are some of the conditions:

• Recent alterations in electrocardiograms or a recent myocardial infarction

• Arrhythmias that are uncontrollable

• Angina pectoris

• Heart block of the third degree

• Sudden and progressive heart failure

Other conditions may exclude exercise on a case-by-case basis and should not be undertaken unless medical consent is obtained. These are some of the conditions:

• High blood pressure

• Cardiomyopathy (heart disease)

• Heart valve disease

• Ventricular ectopy that is complex

• Metabolic illness that is uncontrolled.

CONCLUSION

Even without hormones, women can have a high quality of life following menopause. According to research, postmenopausal women who participate in a complete fitness programme benefit from keeping a healthy physique, bone density levels, and good mental health. Exercise can help reduce osteoporosis, the most common disease among older women. A moderate exercise regimen not only keeps the weight in line, but it also minimizes the risk of stress, anxiety, and depression, all of which are common during and after menopause. Exercise increases muscle mass, strength, balance, and coordination. As a result, unlike medical treatment, workouts work on multiple elements of one's health at the same time. However, the function of exercise in hot flashes remains unclear.

PART 3: EMOTIONAL WELL-BEING: CULTIVATING INNER RESILIENCE

Addressing mood swings, anxiety, and depression during menopause

Menopause and mood swings. Few scientific research back up the notion that menopause causes clinical depression, severe anxiety, or erratic behaviour. Most women get through menopause without having a significant mood issue.

At the same time, hormonal fluctuations, life stresses, disturbed sleep due to night sweats, and concerns about body image, infertility, and ageing can all create mental anguish, leading to mood swings or, in more severe cases depression? Around the time of menopause, many women feel symptoms of depression, stress, worry, and a diminished sense of well-being. This is not surprising given that the end of fertility and the physical changes of midlife may cause women to reflect on their mortality and question the meaning and direction of their lives, as well as whether they have enough children. Those who desired but were unable to have a child may find menopause to be an extremely sad or distressing time.

Mood alterations have been observed in up to 23% of peri- and postmenopausal women in studies. Furthermore, regardless of whether or not symptoms of depression are present, symptoms of anxiety—tension, uneasiness, panic, and worry—are reported more commonly during perimenopause than before it. A sexual dysfunction can be both the cause and the outcome of depression.

Depression, mood, and sex are all factors to consider. The connection between sexuality and depression or emotional state is frequently convoluted. A sexual dysfunction can be both the cause and the outcome of depression. A woman's lack of desire, for example, may contribute to her sadness, but she may also view her desire fall as a result of depression. Furthermore, mood influences emotion, which influences relationship troubles, which has ramifications for sex.

Although the most common sexual side effect of depression or anxiety is decreased desire, other aspects of sexuality can also be affected. When depression is present, orgasm may be more difficult to reach in women. As much as half of SSRI patients report some form of sexual dysfunction.

Antidepressant medicines have sexual side effects. Women suffering from mild to severe depression or anxiety are frequently administered SSRIs (selective serotonin reuptake inhibitors). Although SSRIs are frequently beneficial in treating depression or anxiety, many women (and men) experience sexual adverse effects such as decreased sexual desire, difficulties establishing and sustaining arousal, and problems achieving orgasm. Many people who use SSRIs, such as fluoxetine (Prozac), sertraline (Zoloft), paroxetine (Paxil), and Celexa (citalopram), report some sexual dysfunction.

The good news is that there are options for patients suffering from depression or anxiety whose sex life has been harmed by SSRI therapy. Several non-SSRI antidepressants, such as bupropion (Wellbutrin) and duloxetine (Cymbalta), are less likely to produce sexual dysfunction, and in some women, bupropion has been shown to boost sexual drive and arousal. Furthermore, previous antidepressant drug groups such as tricyclic antidepressants and monoamine oxidase (MAO) inhibitors have not been linked to sexual dysfunction, although they do have other potentially dangerous side effects. New antidepressants, such as vilazodone (Viibryd), are being released and their effect on sexual function must be monitored.

Another alternative is to lessen the dose of your SSRI in the hopes of removing the sexual adverse effects while maintaining the therapy benefits for depression or anxiety. However, this is a difficult balancing act, and any modifications in antidepressant therapy or dosing should be made only after consulting with your healthcare physician.

Self-care and stress-management practices should be practiced.

Self-care has become a trendy topic in recent years, but not everyone understands what it means. It's not all about pampering and spa days. It's all about putting your own mental and physical wellbeing first. Self-care becomes even more crucial when going through menopause or dealing with unexpected life situations. We've come up with 8 techniques to practice self-care throughout menopause to boost your overall wellness.

1.Consume a Nutrient-Rich Diet Getting the correct vitamins, minerals, and other nutrients from the foods we eat is just as crucial during menopause as it has always been. Paying attention to your diet and choosing healthy food choices should be part of practicing self-care throughout menopause.

Consume a diverse diet of nutritious foods rich in lean protein, calcium, and vitamin D. Avoid refined sugary meals and restrict alcohol consumption (which can also cause hot flashes in some women). Because some women struggle with menopausal weight gain, they may need to consider weight management while making dietary decisions.

2. Get moving when it comes to self-care, exercise should be at the top of your list. Physical activity has a plethora of advantages that can help you feel your best during perimenopause and menopause. It relieves stress, provides energy, increases strength, promotes restful sleep, and is a key aspect of weight management. All of these factors are crucial during the perimenopause and menopausal years. Exercise may also help menopausal women avoid osteoporosis. Women should engage in at least 30 minutes of physical activity most days of the week, according to the Office on Women's Health.

3. Look for Ways to Stay Cool

Hot flashes are one of the most prevalent perimenopause and menopausal symptoms that interfere with daily life. Finding strategies to stay cool is a fantastic way to practice self-care throughout menopause. You will feel better mentally when you are more physically comfortable.

Choose breathable textiles like cotton and wear in light layers so you can modify if you get too hot. Some women advise purchasing a portable fan to take to work or use in public places where you don't have control over the temperature. If hot flashes are interfering with your everyday life, consult your doctor about treatment options.

4. Maintain Hydration

Another fantastic technique to practice self-care during menopause is to drink plenty of water. Drinking cold water does more than just chill you down; it also helps your body maintain its temperature. Staying hydrated will also help to alleviate symptoms such as bloating and dryness.

5. Go outside.

Getting outside is beneficial to both our mental and physical wellness. Even those who aren't particularly "outdoorsy" can benefit from spending 30 minutes or so outside. Fresh air may be energizing, and receiving enough vitamin D from sunlight is essential for physical health. You can enjoy the outdoors by jogging or gardening outside.

6. Make an effort to get enough sleep

Getting enough sleep is essential for overall health and wellness. The National Sleep Foundation advises 7 to 9 hours of sleep per night for most adults. During perimenopause and menopause, however, symptoms such as night sweats can make sleeping difficult. While you should consult your doctor about controlling symptoms that cause sleep disturbances, there are other activities you can take to increase your chances of obtaining adequate sleep. Stop using electronic devices such as phones and computers at least 30 minutes before bedtime. Make your sleeping surroundings as comfortable as possible, and wear cool, breathable sleepwear.

7. Maintain Contact with Others

Staying connected to loved ones is a cornerstone of self-care at any time. Make an effort to maintain contact with friends and family. As part of their self-care routine, both extroverts and introverts require some form of human connection. If you are unable to meet in person, text, call, or plan video chats.

8. Consult Your Menopause Specialist

Talking to a doctor about your symptoms is one of the finest strategies to practice self-care throughout menopause. An OB/GYN or reproductive endocrinologist who specializes in menopause care can assist you in managing and preventing symptoms. They can prescribe antidepressants and nutritional supplements.

PART 4: REDISCOVERING YOUR PASSION: EMBRACING NEW BEGINNINGS

Reflecting on personal goals and aspirations during menopause

Setting goals offers you a purpose and a sense of direction. So, as we progress into perimenopause, when those hormones begin to fluctuate and begin to diminish, we can become more self-conscious. This dip in hormones contributes to you feeling more worried, and you carry more stress with you. Those female cuddling hormones may have changed, you may be feeling different, and your emphasis may have shifted. That is very natural and can happen at any time in life. The first recommendation, especially when the hormones are in such a state of flux, is to look at the big picture. Consider the biggest image you can. It's not easy when your hormones are telling you otherwise. For this activity, remove the hormones from the equation, grab a piece of paper, your planner, and a diary, and brainstorm everything you want your life to be. Yes, be self-centered and make it all about you.

Once you've established the big vision, consider what resources you'll need to get there. That may be your financial situation, your home, or your car; list all of the resources you require to achieve that one huge goal. Are they on the same page? Can you achieve your one major goal with the resources you have?

You must then learn to work on yourself. Examine your self-control. The change in hormone profile that occurs during perimenopause and continues into menopause produces a significant alteration in our health. When our female hormones drop, our bone density changes, we experience more aches and pains, we are more prone to migraines, do I need to go on? When these hormones begin to fluctuate, we must pay special attention to our mental health and how we feel about ourselves. Because of the hormonal changes, you may feel more exhausted and fatigued, which may make you feel more self-conscious. This can make you feel even more anxious about what's going on, especially when those hormones are contributing to it! As we progress through perimenopause and into menopause, we must recognize how changes in our hormone profile might affect our physical and emotional health; to do so, we can practice self-mastery.

Finally, one of our main four aims is to examine how you connect and communicate with those around you. How will your objectives impact your relationships? They can be personal, family, or friend relationships, or they can be professional partnerships. Remember that your career may change because of how you feel about yourself at this time; nearly 40% of women throughout the menopausal transition change occupations, jobs, or just leave the workforce. You must address this issue and consider how perimenopause hormones affect what you can and want to accomplish with those around you.

Examine your objectives, and consider whether they are long-term or short-term. What you want out of life and how you want your life to appear, and then take action. This transition into menopause is life-changing for many women, so make it the life you want.

Investigating creative channels and hobbies for self-expression

As a woman who has gone through the changing journey of menopause, I want to share my own experience and observations in order to shed light on this frequently misunderstood stage of life. Menopause, the time between perimenopause and menopause, is a distinct stage with its own set of delights and problems. I hope that by sharing my story, I will inspire and empower other women who are navigating this wonderful, often baffling, but ultimately liberating stage of life.

Accepting Change:

For years, I had heard of menopause and its symptoms, but menopause seemed foreign to me. As I approached my forties, I began to notice changes in my menstrual cycle, hot flashes, and mood swings. It was then that I realized I was at the menopause stage, a natural shift marked by a progressive drop in reproductive hormones.

The physical changes in my body were one of the most visible features of menopause. Hormonal changes caused unpredictable intervals of lighter to heavier flow. Hot flashes, nocturnal sweats, and occasional sleep disruptions became a regular part of my day. These changes were frightening at first, but I soon saw they were a testament to my body's toughness and adaptability.

I used a comprehensive strategy that included physical, emotional, and mental well-being to traverse the menopause journey with grace and self-care. Here are a few strategies that have helped me in my personal journey:

1. Physical Vitality Maintenance:

Exercise became an important part of my menopause experience. Yoga, brisk walking, and dance, for example, not only helped me lose weight and improve my cardiovascular health, but they also provided an outlet for emotional release and self-expression. To boost general vitality, I also focused on eating a balanced diet rich in fruits, vegetables, whole grains, and lean proteins.

2. Compassion for Oneself and Emotional Well-Being:

Accepting self-compassion and nurturing emotional well-being became critical components of my menopause journey. I gave myself permission to feel and process the gamut of emotions that surfaced throughout this period. Journaling, mindfulness practice, and seeking support from loved ones all assisted me in navigating the emotional rollercoaster with greater ease. Embracing self-care habits such as warm baths, meditation, and participating in hobbies that brought me joy was critical to keeping emotional stability.

3. Empowerment and Education:

Learning about menopause was crucial in helping me understand the changes I was going through. I consumed literature, went to seminars, and participated in online forums where women shared their stories. Armed with knowledge, I became an advocate for my own health, holding open discussions with healthcare experts to make informed decisions regarding hormone therapy or other supporting measures.

4. Community and connection:

Surrounding myself with a supportive network of other women going through menopause was crucial to my journey. Joining support groups, going to women's circles, or finding online networks provided a secure area to share stories, seek advice, and offer support. During this transitional period, the power of connection and shared wisdom cannot be overlooked.

5. Accepting Self-Discovery:

Menopause provided me with a once-in-a-lifetime opportunity for self-discovery and personal improvement. I discovered new passions, explored creative outlets, and pursued interests that had been on the backburner for years as I let go of societal expectations and accepted my genuine self. This time in my life allowed me to rediscover my purpose, nourish my spirit, and assert my authority as a knowledgeable and experienced woman.

Conclusion:

The menopause journey is an intensely personal and unique experience. It is a time of self-discovery and exploration.

Menopause without a pill

1. Consume calcium and vitamin D-rich meals.

Menopausal hormonal fluctuations can cause bone weakness, increasing the risk of osteoporosis.

Because calcium and vitamin D are linked to bone health, it's critical to acquire enough of these minerals in your diet.

Adequate vitamin D intake after menopause is also linked to a lower incidence of hip fractures caused by weak bones.

Many foods include calcium, including dairy products such as yoghurt, milk, and cheese.

Green, leafy foods namely kale, collard greens, and spinach which are high in calcium. It's also found in tofu, beans, sardines, and a variety of others.

Calcium-fortified foods, such as specific cereals, fruit juice, or milk substitutes, are also good sources.

Because your skin creates vitamin D when exposed to sunlight, it is your primary source of vitamin D. However, as you age, your skin becomes less efficient at producing it.

Oily fish, eggs, cod liver oil, and vitamin D-fortified meals are all good sources.

2. Maintain a healthy weight.

Weight gain is frequent during menopause.

This could be due to a mix of hormone fluctuations, ageing, lifestyle, and heredity.

Excess body fat, particularly around the waist, raises the risk of acquiring ailments including heart disease and diabetes.

Furthermore, body weight may influence menopausal symptoms.

According to one study of 17,473 postmenopausal women, those who reduced at least 10 pounds (4.5 kg) or 10% of their body weight over a year were more likely to eradicate hot flashes and night sweats (5Trusted Source).

Achieving and maintaining a healthy weight can help with menopause symptoms and illness prevention.

3. Consume plenty of fruits and veggies.

A diet high in fruits and vegetables helps prevent many other menopausal symptoms.

Fruits and vegetables are low in calories and so, helps you feel full, making them ideal for weight loss and maintenance.

They may also aid in the prevention of a variety of disorders, including heart disease (6Trusted Source).

This is significant because the risk of heart disease increases after menopause. This could be attributed to ageing, weight gain, or possibly lower oestrogen levels.

Finally, fruits and vegetables may assist in the prevention of bone loss.

A diet high in fruits and vegetables may help maintain bone health while also preventing weight gain and some disorders.

4. Avoid eating trigger foods.

Certain meals have been linked to hot flashes, nocturnal sweats, and mood swings.

When consumed at night, they may be significantly more likely to be triggers.

Caffeine, alcohol, and sweet or spicy foods are common causes.

Maintain a symptom diary. If you believe that certain foods are causing your menopause symptoms, attempt to limit your intake or avoid them entirely.

Certain meals and beverages listed below causes hot flashes, nocturnal sweats, and mood swings. Caffeine, alcohol, and sweet or spicy foods are examples of this.

5. Exercise on a regular basis.

Currently, there is insufficient evidence to determine if exercise is useful in treating hot flashes and night sweats (8Trusted Source, 9Trusted Source).

Other benefits of regular exercise, such as Pilates-based exercise programmes, are supported by studies. These advantages include increased energy and metabolism, healthier joints and bones, reduced stress, and greater sleep.

A study in Korea, for example, found that a 12-week walking fitness programme enhanced physical and mental health, as well as general quality of life in a group of 40 menopausal women.

Regular physical activity has also been linked to improved general health and protection against diseases and conditions such as cancer, heart disease, stroke, high blood pressure, type 2 diabetes, obesity, and osteoporosis (13Trusted Source).

Menopausal women have an increased risk of heart disease; however, numerous studies suggest that regular exercise may help minimize this risk (14Trusted Source, 15).

Regular exercise helps improve menopausal symptoms such as insomnia, anxiety, depression, and exhaustion. It can also help to prevent weight gain and a variety of ailments and conditions.

6. Consume more phytoestrogen-rich foods.

Phytoestrogens are plant chemicals that naturally occur and can mimic the actions of oestrogen in the body.

As a result, they may aid in hormone balance.

The substantial use of phytoestrogens in Asian countries such as Japan is suggested to explain why menopausal women in these countries rarely have hot flashes.

Phytoestrogen-rich foods include:

• Soybeans and soy-based goods

• Tofu

• Tempeh.

• Linseeds

• Flaxseeds

• Toasted sesame seeds

• Beans

However, the phytoestrogen concentration of foods varies depending on how they are processed.

One study discovered that soy-rich diets were associated with lower cholesterol levels, blood pressure, and the severity of hot flashes and nocturnal sweats in women approaching menopause (16Trusted Source).

However, the argument over whether soy products are healthy or hazardous for health persists.

Evidence suggests that natural phytoestrogen sources are superior to supplements or processed diets with additional soy protein.

Phytoestrogen-rich foods may offer minor benefits for hot flashes and heart disease risk. However, the evidence is conflicting.

7. Drink plenty of water.

Dryness is a common problem during menopause. This is most likely caused by a drop in oestrogen levels.

These symptoms can be lifted by drinking 8 to 12 glasses of water every day.

Drinking water also helps to minimize bloating caused by hormonal changes.

Furthermore, water can assist prevent weight gain and aid in weight loss by making you feel full and somewhat improving your metabolism (19Trusted Source, 20Trusted Source).

Drinking 17 ounces (500 ml) of water 30 minutes before a meal may result in 13% fewer calories consumed during the meal.

8. Reduce your intake of refined sugar and processed meals.

Diets strong in processed carbohydrates and sugar can produce blood sugar spikes and drops, leaving you weak and irritable. This may aggravate menopausal physical and mental symptoms.

In fact, one study discovered that high-refined-carbohydrate diets may raise the incidence of depression in postmenopausal women.

Diets heavy in processed foods may also have an impact on bone health, particularly if these items replace the nutrients you require from a regular balanced diet.

A large observational study indicated that diets heavy in processed and snack foods were associated with poor bone quality in women aged 50 to 59 (7Trusted Source).

9. Avoid skipping meals.

Eating on a regular basis may be beneficial during menopause.

Irregular eating patterns might exacerbate certain menopausal symptoms and make weight management more challenging.

Skipping meals was related with 4.3% less weight loss in a yearlong weight management programme for postmenopausal women (22Trusted Source).

10. Consume protein-rich foods.

Eating protein throughout the day can help prevent the aging-related loss of lean muscle mass.

One study discovered that eating protein at each meal throughout the day may slow down muscle loss related to ageing (23).

In addition to preventing muscle loss, high protein diets can aid in weight loss by increasing satiety and increasing the number of calories expended (24Trusted Source).

Protein-rich foods include meat, fish, eggs, beans, nuts, and dairy.

Regular consumption of high-quality protein may help prevent lean muscle loss, aid in weight loss, and regulate mood and sleep.

11. Utilize natural supplements.

Many women may explore using natural goods and therapies to alleviate the symptoms of menopause.

However, the evidence for many of these is weak.

The following are the most commonly used natural supplements for minimizing menopausal symptoms:

Phytoestrogens. These can be obtained from natural foods or supplementation. There is currently insufficient data to recommend them for symptom relief during menopause

Cohosh (black cohosh). Although some studies have suggested that black cohosh can help with hot flashes, the evidence is conflicting. Furthermore, long-term data on the safety of this supplement is lacking

The red clover. According to a review of studies, red clover isoflavone supplements may help reduce the daily frequency of hot flashes from three per day to one per day. The study authors did warn, however, that additional specific research is needed to confirm the effects of red clover on decreasing flushing episodes and other menopausal symptoms (29).

Additional supplements. More research is needed to determine the efficacy of additional commonly used supplements such probiotics, prebiotics, cranberry extract, kava, DHEA-S, dong quai, and evening primrose oil in alleviating menopause symptoms like hot flashes and night sweats (30, 31Trusted Source).

Frequently Asked Questions about Natural Menopause Remedies

How can I balance my hormones naturally throughout menopause?

Regular exercise and a nutrient-dense diet can aid in hormone balance throughout menopause. To treat symptoms, you may also need to take supplements or drugs in some circumstances. Consult your doctor to determine what you require for menopause symptoms.

What are some natural menopausal remedies?

Herbal supplements are natural solutions for menopause symptoms. Some of these contain phytoestrogens, which are plant estrogen that aid in the balance of low hormone levels during menopause. They may help with symptoms such as hot flashes and nocturnal sweats.

It's crucial to keep in mind that even over-the-counter vitamins can be effective and interact with other prescriptions. Before you begin taking supplements, consult with your doctor to ensure that they are safe for you.

What foods aggravate menopause?

Foods that raise your blood sugar (glucose) levels can exacerbate some menopausal symptoms. Refined, processed carbohydrates, such as sweet and starchy foods such as:

- ➢ cookies
- ➢ chips
- ➢ cracker
- ➢ White flour-based baked foods
- ➢ Limit your intake of fried meals as well.

Skipping meals or eating meals low in protein and natural fats can further exacerbate menopausal symptoms.

Conclusion

Menopause affects all women at some point in their lives. Individual menopausal experiences vary greatly, and how women choose to manage their menopause will be determined by a variety of factors, including age at menopause, the presence of any symptoms, and how these influence their quality of life. Their decisions will also be influenced by risk factors for cardiovascular disease, cancer, and osteoporosis. Some women prefer a more "natural" approach to menopause care, while others opt for hormone replacement therapy (HRT).

Dietary and lifestyle changes are helpful for all women, especially during the menopausal years, for minimizing symptoms, enhancing general well-being, and lowering the risk of health issues. As part of menopausal treatment, women should ensure that they get enough exercise and eat a healthy, well-balanced diet.

www.ingramcontent.com/pod-product-compliance
Lightning Source LLC
Chambersburg PA
CBHW071100260726

48661CB00006B/2366